Our appreciation
for your time
and wonderful
presentation

Nigel Steel

I thought you
might especially like P.23,
177

All the Alternatives to Aging Are Bad

Thoughts on Growing Older

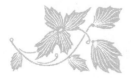

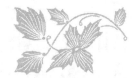

All the Alternatives to Aging Are Bad

Thoughts on Growing Older

by
R. Knight Steel, M.D.

illustrations by
Jim Harris

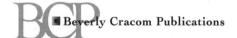

BCP ■ **Beverly Cracom Publications**

St. Louis, MO • **Wilton, CT** • **Pasadena, CA**

A joint venture between Beverly Foundation and Cracom Publishing, Inc.

Neither the publisher nor the author intend that this book be used in lieu of appropriate medical care. Decisions about using the information provided here are entirely at the reader's discretion. Every person should have a physician who can advise that person as to the merits of following any recommendation in this book, either expressed or implied.

Library of Congress Cataloging-in-Publication Data
All the alternatives to aging are bad: thoughts on
   growing older/ [collected] by R. Knight Steel.
         p.   cm.
  ISBN 1-886657-03-3
  1. Old age—Quotations, maxims, etc. 2. Aging—
Quotations, maxims, etc. I. Steel, R. Knight.
PN6084.05A45 1996
305.26—dc20   95-25083
                                CIP

During my years as a practicing physician in Boston, I made hundreds of home visits to elders. This book consists of bits of wisdom gleaned from conversations I had with these wonderful people over the years.

It is my hope that by reading these thoughts you will be able to more fully appreciate, accept and even embrace the phenomenon of aging.

This book is dedicated to all who are aging, which is to say all of us.

It is also dedicated to my wife and children with whom I have been privileged to spend my period of aging.

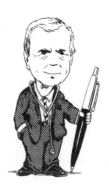

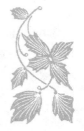

Contents

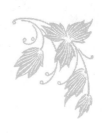

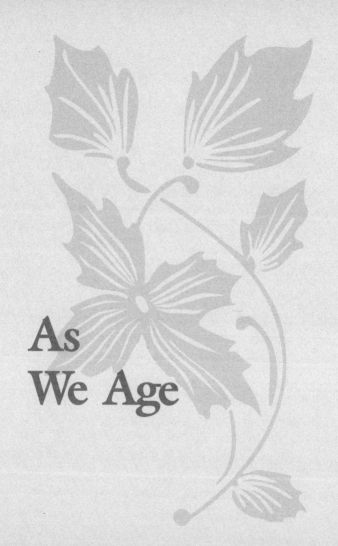

As
We Age

All things age
not just you.

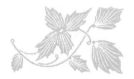

Aging, for many,
seems to be experienced
in bursts of time
rather than as a
continuous process.

If you are over 50
you are part of the
most rapidly growing
segment of the population.

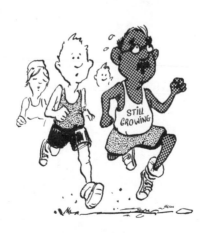

65

isn't a natural milestone.

It's a manmade marker
chosen by those wishing to
implement policy.

If you had lived
400 years ago,
you might have been
a model for one of
Rembrandt's paintings
of that society's
elders.

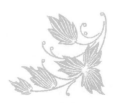

To be "mature"
doesn't mean to be
"overripe."

If you have made it
this far in life,
you surely have
a lot going for you.

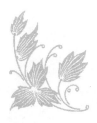

No matter what our age,
old isn't "them"
it's "us"
in the future.

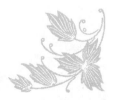

Matters
of Health

Just when I thought
genetics would have
little to offer me,
scientists have begun
to discover genetically
determined
risk factors
for the diseases
of old age.

Having one or more
chronic illnesses
is the norm
for those past 50!

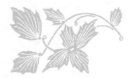

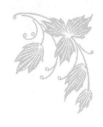

Many illnesses,
no matter where
they are centered in the body,
may begin with confusion.

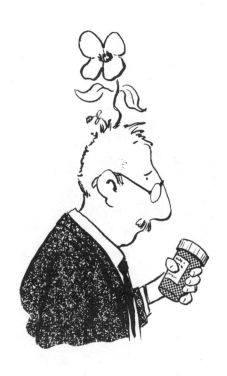

Most medications
have more than one effect
on the body.

Many diseases
are not curable
but most
are manageable.

For many
a functional inability,
addressing just one of
the causes of it
may diminish
or even eliminate it.

Function can often
be maintained,
or only minimally
compromised,
even when cure
is not possible.

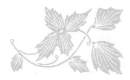

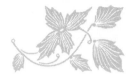

With the rapid advances
in science and medicine,
formerly untreatable diseases
now may have
treatment options.

Innovative technology
can often
assist the disabled
even when
drugs and surgery
cannot.

At least until
very late in life,
aging rarely diminishes
the capacity for
most routine activity.

Disability
isn't the same as
inability.

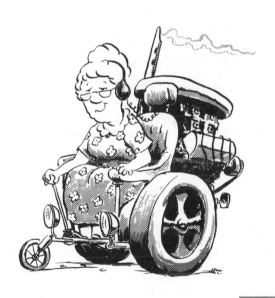

As a general rule,
increasing age
requires
a more detailed assessment
of health, function and
quality of life when
any medical treatment
is considered.

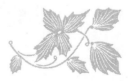

Always seek information pertinent to health from the best scientific sources. Write them, phone them, "e-mail" them.

Choose a physician
who is concerned
not only with
the diagnosis and treatment
of your disease
but also with
your ability to function.

Review all possible
medical options
and then ask your doctor
what he or she would do
if confronted with a
similar set of circumstances
and why.

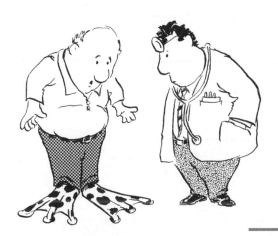

A physician should be
competent and sympathetic
not just one
or the other.

No matter what the number of individual medical specialists in the "orchestra," one "conductor" is required.

Symptoms
under everyday
circumstances
are infrequently due to
the process of aging.

Any regimen of medication
too complicated to follow
is just that–too complicated.

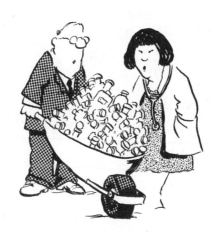

Ask your doctor
to simplify your program.

When considering
elective surgery,
take into account
the duration of
the recovery period
as well as
the risks of
the procedure.

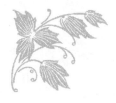

Recovery periods
tend to lengthen
as we age.

When rehabilitative
procedures
seem repetitive
and tedious,
remind yourself that
even Olympic athletes
complain during training.

As hospitals are not
always "hospitable,"
go there if you need to
and don't if you don't.

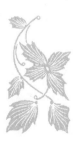

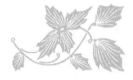

It's wise
to prepare for death,
but not to the point of
its being an obsession.

People often find it
reassuring to write out
an advance directive,
or living will,
detailing their wishes
should they be too ill
to participate in their own
health care decisions.

I've always had difficulty
understanding the phrase
"terminal illness"
because
we are all terminal
it's just
a matter of degree!

Planning
for
the Future

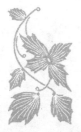

The human animal
is robust.

By the year 2025
there will be
over 1 billion
elderly human animals
worldwide.

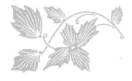

Consider the future,
as you will most likely
live to experience it.

It's essential
to plan ahead
no matter what your age.
Most of us
will be here
for a while longer.

Planning every detail
of the retirement years
isn't necessary.

But considering
some aspects of this period
well in advance
is almost always beneficial.

It may be
especially traumatic
to relocate immediately upon
retirement.

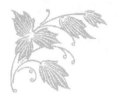

Today
is the best time
to consider ways
to ensure
your independence
tomorrow.

Guilt must
be a form of
capital investment.
It often continues
to accumulate interest
over the years.

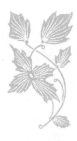

It seems impossible
to predict
the worth of things.
Just look at penny stamps and
baseball cards.

Prevention

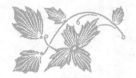

It is regretable
that it seems more exciting
to recount
one's illnesses
and treatments
than to
describe one's plans
for health
maintenance.

Preventive health care,
not as apt to
make as many headlines
as death and disease,
quietly offers
substantial benefits
to people of all ages
even the very old.

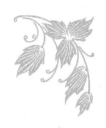

Fitness training
may improve
muscle strength
even in those
80 and above.

The best diet
to promote health
over a lifetime
is still
under discussion.

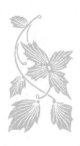

If your mother
always told you
to eat your vegetables because
they were
good for you
she probably was right.

Although
caloric requirements
usually decline with age,
that is no reason
why food
can't be prepared
to satisfy
both body and soul!

Be aware of
the pills you pop
as much as you are of
the food you eat!

Many preventive
health measures
begun in early adulthood
are the retirement plans
for well-being.

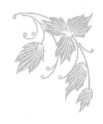

Supplements
to retirement resources
don't necessarily
have to be in cash.

Saving for retirement
means banking
not only money
but also
bone and muscle.

Long-term management
is a good strategy
for your physical well-being
as well as
for your financial assets.

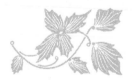

Prevention means
not only
"preventing" illness
for all time,
but also
"delaying"
the onset of disease
and functional disability.

Rainy Day
Support

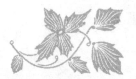

When planning
for a "rainy day"
anticipate other setbacks
besides financial ones.
Disabilities
that restrict mobility
may also
require consideration.

Regrettably
we are rarely able
to schedule an illness
for a time
when business is slow
or our children
are available.

A support system
should be designed
to meet a need.

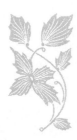

Many families
are willing to be
as helpful as possible
in the care of
an older relative,
even when their own
day-to-day responsibilities
place other demands
on their
time and energy.

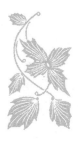

Caring for a loved one
who is ill
is a uniquely
exhausting task.

Most people find
that by arranging
for some assistance
in the care of a loved one,
they can provide that care
for a longer period of time.

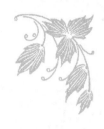

Even people
who are
dependent upon others
can provide support.

Most communities
have an assortment
of home-delivered services
ranging from
Chinese dinners
to professional health care.

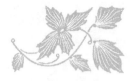

All right,
I agree, as a rule
service
isn't what it used to be!

When making a decision
about a significant issue,
do so with the future
of loved ones in mind.

Form
and Function

Getting up from a chair
requires not only
that the person have
a measure
of functional ability
but also that the chair
be properly designed.

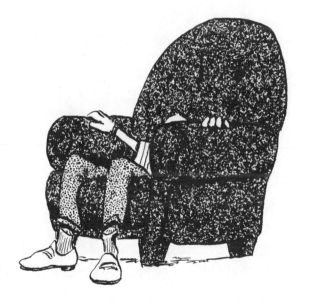

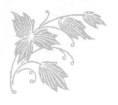

Aging
results in
increasing variability,
both in terms of
life experiences
and physiologic functions.

Because aging results in
slowed reaction times,
card sharks
may be in more trouble
as they get older!

Failing eyesight, associated with aging, can often be corrected or arrested.

It is commonplace
for all persons,
but especially those
past middle age,
to have difficulty with vision
when directly facing
a bright light.

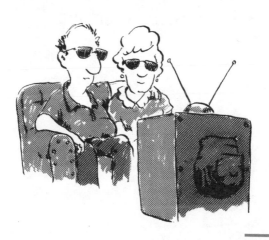

I have always believed
that sharks are more advanced
than humans
for, reportedly,
they simply grow new teeth
when others wear out.

Most persons
lose some
sense of smell
with age.

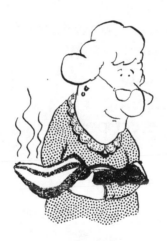

This can be good or bad
depending on the circumstance!

Given the prevalence
of low back pain,
one has to wonder whether
the human animal
was ever intended
to assume
the erect posture!

With age,
your body is less able
to adapt to
extremes of temperature.

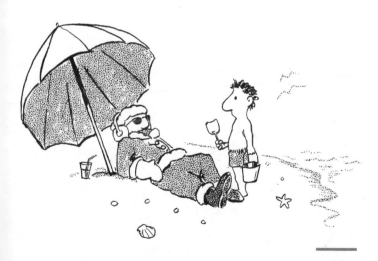

Assistance with
personal hygiene and
intimate bodily functions
is an ordinary occurrence
for most people
at some time in their lives.

Incontinence may be
eliminated or helped
with medical treatment.

Depression isn't uncommon in older persons, and therefore symptoms of depression warrant evaluation.

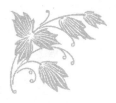

If hearing loss is causing
the quality of your life
to decrease,
a hearing aid may benefit more
than just your hearing.

Emphasizing consonants
and lowering the pitch
of the voice
may help someone
with a hearing disability
to understand.

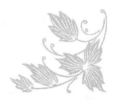

Many people talking at once
results not in
many opinions being heard
but in none being understood.

It's not just
because you're older
that people don't
listen to you
most people don't listen
to others
no matter what their age.

Aging doesn't
seem to make it any easier
to admit we're wrong
at least for most of us!

Review your habits
on a regular basis
and make adjustments
if needed!

Older persons
should give up smoking
not only because
it is harmful,
but also because
they are role models
for youth.

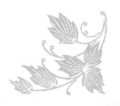

Alcohol is
tolerated less well
with age.

Driving when impaired
by alcohol or drugs
is foolish at any age.

Standing up abruptly after a large meal may result in lightheadedness leading to a fall.

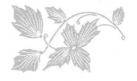

A sudden
burst of exertion
may lead to injury.

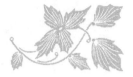

Pamper your joints.

Develop a foot fetish
because there are
few parts of your body
that will be more important to
you over time.

Because the
"rhythm" of stairs
varies according to
the height and depth
of each step, some stairs
are easier to climb than others.

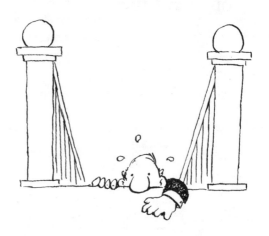

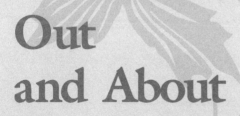

Out
and About

Just as our
living environment
was important to each of us
when we were young,
so it is as we grow older.

Place
frequently used items
at a height
that's easy to reach.

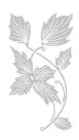

Accidents,
one of the greatest
causes of disability
in older persons,
are frequently preventable.

Play it safe.
Install grab bars in the tub,
have emergency numbers
handy and keep
stairways well lit.

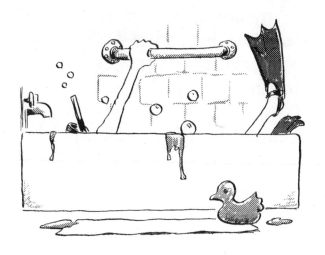

Why not
listen to the advice
so frequently given
to children?

Leave yourself enough time!

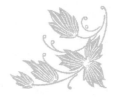

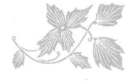

If you can't see
where you're going,
don't go.

Difficulties with walking
should be addressed
as soon as possible
before they contribute
to falling,
or such a fear of falling,
that mobility becomes
unduly restricted.

Stylish shoes
need not impair balance.

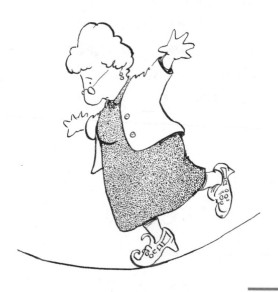

Have to circulate
at a social function?
Make sure your garters
are not so tight that
they prevent your blood from
circulating as well.

Even for a short distance, take
the time
to turn around
and walk forward
rather than
trying to save time
by walking backward.

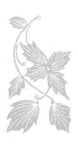

Some falls
are a direct result
of trying,
just this once,
to carry too many packages.

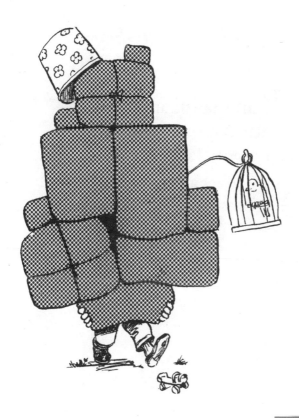

Being familiar
with your surroundings
prevents falls.

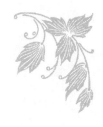

It is fine to
fall in love with a pet,
but hardly desirable
to fall over one!

For some,
plants are
as enjoyable as pets
and they cost less to feed!

Age and Youth

People of all ages
may fail to appreciate
the benefits of their age.

There is a freedom
that comes with age
as many of the
responsibilities
of earlier years
have been met.

"Carefree" youth wasn't necessarily "care free."

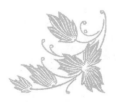

If you think aging is bad,
just consider
what it would be like
to be 15 years of age
for a lifetime!

"Acting your age"
at any age
really means
appreciating
your capabilities
and accepting
your limitations.

Whining about one's age,
often attributed
to the elderly,
is a trait most common,
in my experience,
to those
between the ages
of 12 and 16!

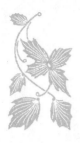

I doubt
I could live long enough
to "grow up"
in all respects!

Being "eccentric"
is in vogue
at any age!

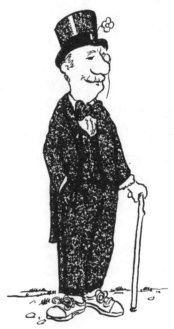

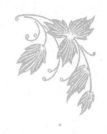

Being "macho"
is better left
to those
who are younger.

Being set in one's ways
is a trait
more typically displayed
by teenagers
than by older persons!

Generalities about life depend
on what part
of the life span
one is generalizing about.

Stereotypes about youth
do seem to be true
quite often!

Common sense
isn't age-adjusted.

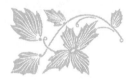

We've all done
truly stupid things
in our lives
and as we age
we have a chance
to do more of them.

Wisdom and experience
are neither synonymous
nor mutually exclusive.

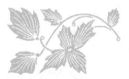

Even a lifetime
of experience
doesn't guarantee
immunity from
con artists and swindlers.

Why are tattered clothes
perceived as hip
on the
younger generation ...

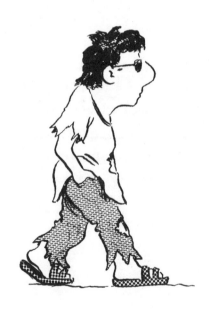

but shabby
on those who are older!

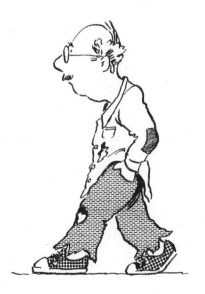

Clothing styles change
over time
affording a
constant source
of amusement.

Thank heavens we seem to have moved beyond the era when "proper" clothing was drab.

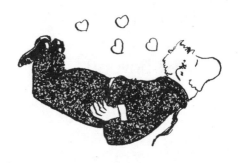

Sexual relationships
in later life
can take on
a breadth and depth
beyond the mere physical.

If cosmetics and fragrances
were only for the young,
manufacturers
of these products
would go out of business!

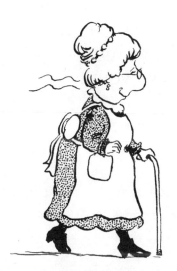

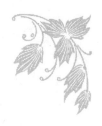

The older generation
has experienced youth,
but youth
has not experienced
old age.

If young people
speak to you
as if you are alien
be reminded
that in many ways you are and
smile knowingly.

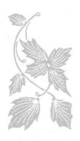

The young have
stories to tell too.
Be a good listener.

It can be difficult
to know when to comment
and when not to,
especially when speaking with
one's offspring!

When dealing with
a difficult person,
try to imagine,
just for a moment,
that the person
is your grandchild!
It may help!

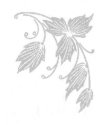

Members of
the older generation
frequently find
common cause
with the
children of their children.

Most of us,
as we age,
wish to live
near our children
but not necessarily
with them.

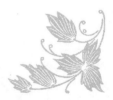

The young
involved in their own lives
may be as unavailable
as we were at their age.

The young of today
won't necessarily have
the same kind of relationship
with their parents
that the older generation had
with theirs.

You needn't
try to solve
every problem
your children
or grandchildren will face
nor even try
to anticipate them.

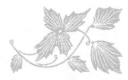

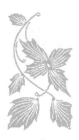

The words
"old" and "young"
are not absolutes.

Education
isn't exclusively
for the young.

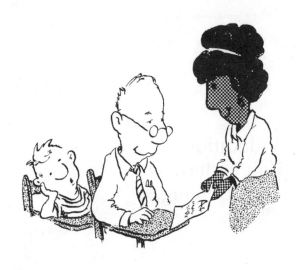

People of any age
can benefit from
becoming educated
about something new.

Although older persons
attending school
may find it uncomfortable
to be surrounded by
persons much their junior,
that shouldn't dissuade them
from enrolling.

For the first time
in history to be old
isn't unusual.

The number
of popular myths
about old age
exceeds
the number
of known truths.

Although the color
"gray" has been associated
with weakness,
this shouldn't necessarily apply
to people
with that color of hair.

There is
an increasing number
of very functional
90 year olds
in our society.

Creativity
isn't the domain
solely of the young.

Numerous examples
in the arts and sciences
attest to this.

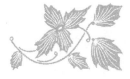

Many of us
don't bloom
until later in life.

Some of
the most famous
works of art
were painted by
persons with failing vision.

Being "too old"
or "too young"
doesn't bar people from
life's accomplishments
and enjoyments.

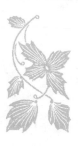

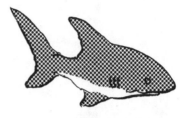

If there has been
one thing
that you have
always wanted to do,

it may not be
too late to do it.

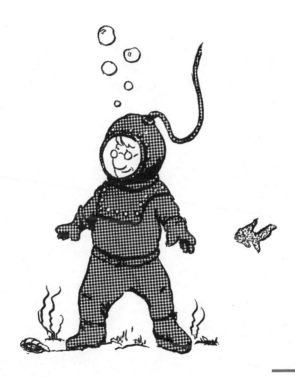

Even Fred Astaire
had to practice
before
he could use a cane
both effectively
and with grace.

Successful aging
suggests something other
than aging
without any changes.

"Renaissance"
is a better word than
"retirement."

In the renaissance
of retirement
many people have
fulfilling experiences
acting on their beliefs.

It's quite acceptable
to take vacations
even when
not employed
the remainder
of the year.

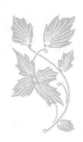

Planning for trips
isn't just
half the fun,
it doubles the fun
by avoiding
potential problems.

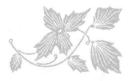

There are
always things
that we wish
we had done differently.
Indeed
this list grows
with the passage of time.

It has always been
"too late"
for some things.

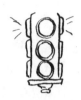

Because there is
no going back
and we can't stand still,
there seems to be
only one direction to go.

You can
keep on rolling
without having to drive.

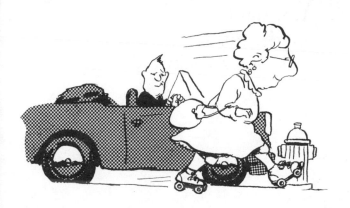

You can't
see the future
by looking backward.

W hat was once
embarrassing
may no longer be so.

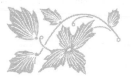

Maybe the reason
some get wiser with age
is because
there is a gene for wisdom
which switches on
at about the age of 50!

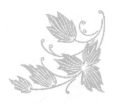

Trees make
wonderful models
in many respects,
but remember
that they add rings
around their middle
as they age!

Have you ever wondered whether older dinosaurs had wrinkles?

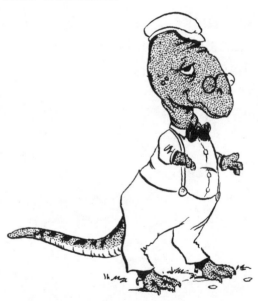

Old
and New

The range of opportunities
for all of us,
not only our children
and grandchildren,
is vastly greater
than in the past.

Although some may believe
that life was "simpler"
a half-century ago,
it was no less risky
and considerably
more limiting.

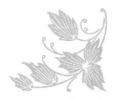

"Commuting" to work
without leaving home
is a much more feasible option
today than even
a few years ago.

Thank heaven
all things
aren't the way
they used to be.

In the past
only a small percentage
of the population
reached old age.

Any one of us
might have been excluded
from that group.

Many things
are just the way
they used to be.

They only seem different
because our perspective
changes with time.

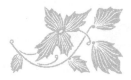

In some ways
we are exactly
who we have always been
and in other ways
we are vastly changed,
molded over time
by our experiences.

Even if
the circumstances
of a situation
closely resemble
those of the past,
your response today
may need to be different.

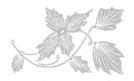

Sometimes it is startling
to recognize
that events of history
recalled with such emotion
by those who
experienced them
are only read about
in history books
by those
a generation younger.

Since the media
sensationalizes violence,
any change
in the morality of man
may be more an impression
than reality.

At times
the speed of change
is so rapid that
after even a short time
circumstances seem altered
almost beyond recognition.

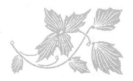

It isn't necessary
to understand the way
all things work
in order to use them.

Don't be fearful
of computers
at least any more
than the rest of us!

For they now allow everyone
even the most infirm
to communicate with
the rest of the world.

User-friendly technology
can be
user-unfriendly
at any age.

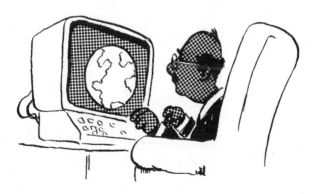

Aging isn't the cause
of failing to understand.

Failure is common
at any age.

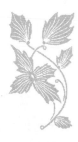

Science continually
invalidates
many of our
long-held beliefs.

At times it is difficult
to remember
that we
always have
been vulnerable
and always will be.

Because holidays
stir up memories,
it's not unusual
to feel a sense of sadness
on these days.

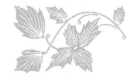

Don't hesitate
to call your
friends and family
frequently.
If you reach them
at an inconvenient moment,
call back.

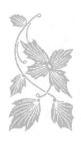

Teatime may be
an especially convenient time
to meet with relatives
and friends of all ages.

It's a good idea
to make new friends.
After all
"old" friends
were once new.

The attitude
of "old" friends
may change
because of new
circumstances
in their lives.

When people age
they don't become either
sweet or mean
they just become older.

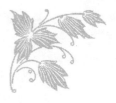

I keep forgetting
why we worry about
our memory so much!

Trouble with memory
is a sure bet
when the past is recalled
only as the
"good old days"!

Not all traditions are good.

Enjoy your
unique journey
through time.